ULTIMATE FATTY LIVER DIET COOKBOOK

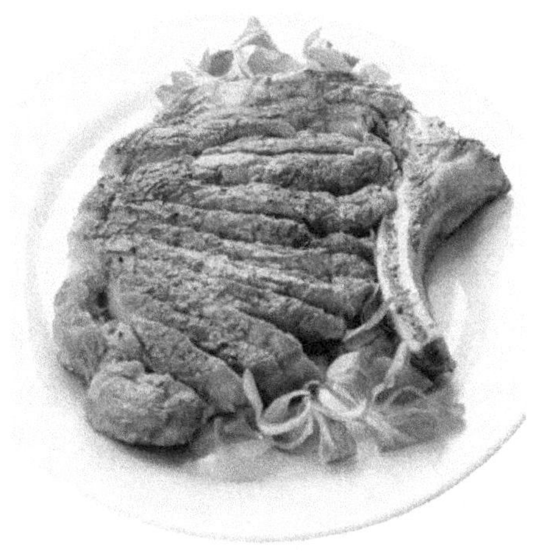

Quick & Easy Delicious Recipes To Cleanse Your Liver

Leroy Johnson

CONTENTS

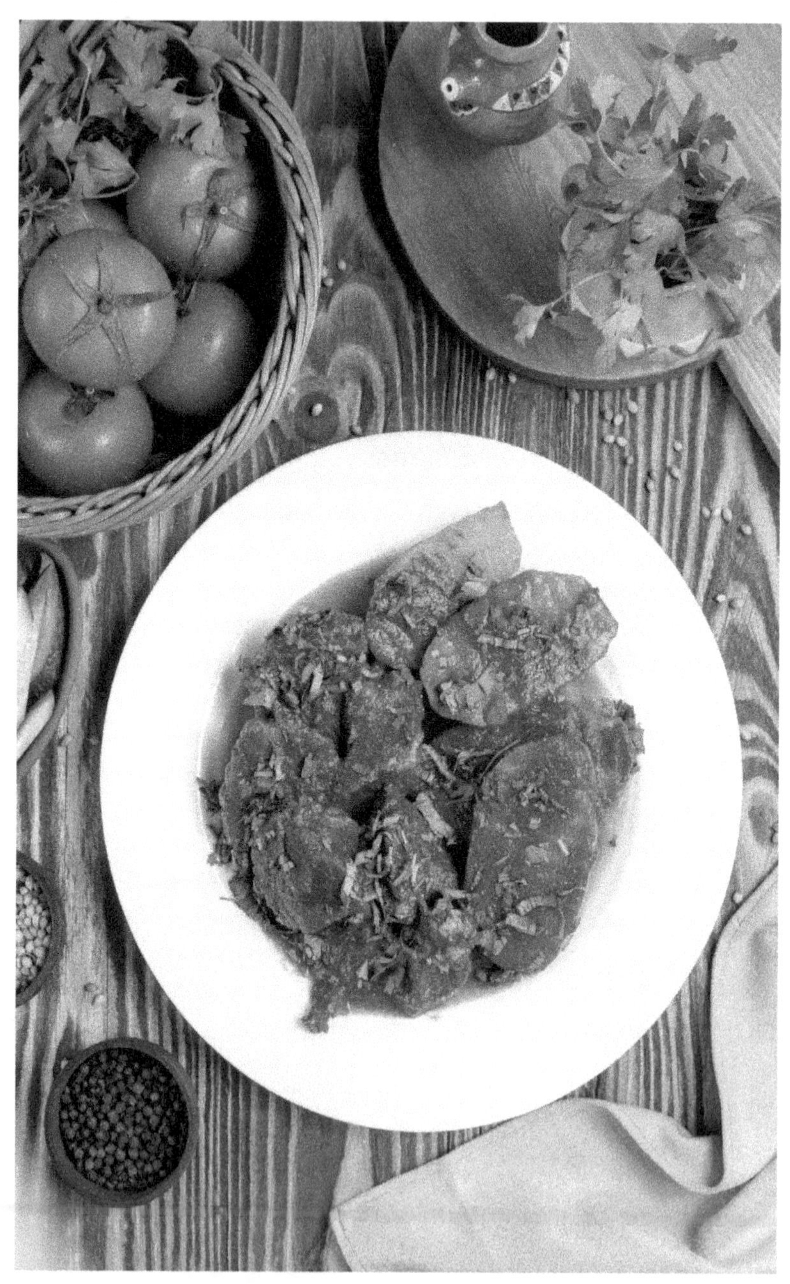

INTRODUCTION

In a peaceful, beautiful town settled in the core of the open country, they carried on with an elderly person named Samuel. Samuel had seen his reasonable part of life's promising and less promising times, however the greatest test he confronted was his battle with liver infection. He had been determined to have a serious instance of liver cirrhosis, a condition that had created a long shaded area over his sundown years.

Samuel's once-dynamic life had been diminished to a delicate presence. His skin had turned a wiped out shade of yellow, and he was ceaselessly exhausted. Strolling even brief distances had turned into a Considerable undertaking. Specialists had given him dreary news - there was no remedy for his condition, and he made some restricted memories left.

Unflinching by the dreary forecast, Samuel left on an excursion to recover his wellbeing. He dove profoundly into research, pouring over innumerable articles and books on liver wellbeing. He found that the liver, a wonderful organ, was able to recover whenever given the right circumstances. With assurance in his heart, Samuel chose to change his eating routine.

His kitchen racks were before long loaded up with a variety of brilliant vegetables and natural products. Samuel embraced a plant-based diet, wealthy in mixed greens, tomatoes, and new berries. Gone were the times of handled food varieties and sweet beverages. He hydrated and supplanted his morning espresso with green tea.

Yet, his eating regimen was just important for the change. Samuel realized that exercise was similarly significant. Despite the fact that he was unable to run long distance races, he began with delicate strolls in the town, step by step expanding the distance. The outside air and the excellence of nature turned into his friends on this recuperating venture.

The weeks transformed into months, and Samuel started to see unpretentious changes. His skin recovered a sound shade, and the dormancy that had held him hostage began to release its grasp. The customary strolls provided him a feeling of motivation and a chance to interface with his kindred locals. He shared his freshly discovered information and motivated numerous to embrace better ways of life.

His advancement was out and out astounding. As his body gradually recuperated, the tests showed that his liver was answering decidedly to his better approach for life. The specialists were bewildered and couldn't really accept what they were seeing. Samuel's liver was recovering, resisting the chances. Expressions of Samuel's marvelous recuperation spread quickly through the town and then some. Individuals made a trip from neighboring towns to meet the one who had switched his liver infection with the force of a straightforward, healthy eating regimen. Samuel's home turned into a center point of trust and motivation. As the seasons changed, Samuel did as well. His once weak casing currently remained steadfast and consistent. His bliss was irresistible, and the town celebrated in his victory over the apparently outlandish chances. Samuel wasn't simply an elderly person who had beaten liver infection; he had turned into an image of versatility and the extraordinary force of a solid way of life.

The town observed Samuel's recuperation with a fantastic gala, and the table was weighed down with an overflow of products of the soil. Samuel, the elderly person who had whenever been informed he had a brief period left, presently remained as a demonstration of the exceptional limit of the human body to recuperate when supported with the ideal decisions.

Thus, in that curious town, a straightforward story of an elderly person and his excursion from sickness to energetic well being became legend. Samuel's inheritance lived on, moving ages to embrace the groundbreaking sorcery of a solid eating routine, demonstrating that it's never past time to pick a superior way and that, occasionally, the right eating regimen can work supernatural occurrences past creative mind.

CHAPTER 1

1.1   What is liver disease?

The liver is an exceptional organ in your body, situated on the right side, just underneath your rib cage. It assumes a vital part in different physical processes, like handling supplements, separating poisons, and managing glucose. Notwithstanding, the liver is helpless to different sicknesses that can disturb it,s not unexpected capabilities. In this 1,000-word article, we will investigate liver illness, its sorts, causes, side effects, and preventive estimates in straightforward English.

1.2   Liver Disease Infection

Liver infection, frequently alluded to as hepatic illness, includes a great many circumstances that influence the liver's design and capability. The liver is a fundamental organ answerable for a few crucial errands, including.

1. **Metabolism:** The liver aides separate and store supplements from the food we eat, similar to carbs, fats, and proteins.

2.**Detoxification**: It channels harmful substances from the blood, eliminating poisons and medications from your body.

3. **Production**: The liver produces proteins fundamental for blood coagulating and controlling cholesterol.

4. **Storage**: It stores glycogen, a wellspring of speedy energy, and fundamental nutrients and minerals.

5. **Bile Production**: The liver produces bile, fundamental for assimilation and the ingestion of fats.

Given its essential job, any aggravation in liver capability can have serious results.

1.3   Types of Liver Disease

Liver infections are ordered into different sorts, each with its one of a kind qualities and causes. The most well-known types include.

1. **Hepatitis**: Hepatitis is the aggravation of the liver and can be brought about by viral diseases, liquor misuse, or certain prescriptions.

2. **Cirrhosis**: Cirrhosis is the scarring of the liver tissue, frequently brought about by constant liquor misuse or viral hepatitis.

3. **Fatty Liver Disease:** This condition is described by an amassing of fat in the liver and can be brought about

by heftiness, diabetes, or unnecessary liquor utilization.

4. **Liver Cancer**: Liver malignant growth can foster in the actual liver (essential liver disease) or spread from different pieces of the body (metastatic liver malignant growth).

5. **Hemochromatosis**: This hereditary issue prompts an exorbitant development of iron in the liver and different organs.

1.4   Causes of Liver Disease

Understanding the reasons for liver sickness is significant for its anticipation. A few normal causes include.

1. **Viral Infections**: Infections like hepatitis A, B, and C can taint the liver and cause irritation, prompting liver illness.

2. **Alcohol Abuse:** Unnecessary and delayed liquor utilization can harm liver cells and result in alcoholic liver illness.

3. **Obesity**: Heftiness is frequently connected with non-alcoholic greasy liver illness (NAFLD), where fat amasses in the liver.

4. **Medications**: A few drugs, particularly when taken in high dosages or over an extensive stretch, can hurt the liver.

5. **Genetics**: Certain hereditary circumstances, similar to hemochromatosis, Wilson's infection, and immune system liver illnesses, can expand the gamble of liver sickness.

6. **Toxins**: Openness to ecological poisons, like modern synthetics or certain natural enhancements, can harm the liver.

1.5   Side effects of Liver Disease

Perceiving the side effects of liver sickness is fundamental for early discovery and therapy. Normal side effects might include.

1. **Jaundice**: Yellowing of the skin and eyes because of the development of bilirubin in the blood.

2. **Fatigue**: An industrious sensation of sleepiness and shortcoming.

3. **Abdominal Pain:** Distress or torment in the upper right half of the mid-region.

4. **Swelling**: Expanding in the mid-region or legs because of liquid maintenance.

5. **Dark Urine:** Pee that is more obscure in variety than expected.

6. **Pale Stools**: Stools that seem pale or earth hued.

7. **Loss of Appetite**: A decreased craving to eat or unexplained weight reduction.

It's vital to note that the seriousness and blend of these side effects can differ contingent upon the kind and phase of liver infection.

1.6   Preventive Measures for Liver Disease

Forestalling liver illness is feasible through basic way of life changes and customary medical services observing. Here are a few preventive measures.

1. **Limit Alcohol**: In the event that you drink liquor, do as such with some restraint. For most grown-ups, this implies depending upon one beverage each day for ladies and up to two beverages each day for men.

2. **Healthy Diet**: Keep a decent eating regimen wealthy in organic products, vegetables, entire grains, and lean proteins. Diminish sugar and soaked fat admission.

3. **Exercise**: Participate in normal actual work to keep a sound weight, as corpulence is a gamble factor for liver illness.

4. **Vaccination**: Receive an immunization shot against hepatitis A and B in the event that you are in danger. This is especially significant for medical care laborers and explorers to high-gamble with regions.

5. **Safe Sex and Hygiene**: Practice safe sex to forestall the transmission of hepatitis B and C. Furthermore, follow great cleanliness practices to forestall hepatitis A.

6. **Medication Awareness**: Be mindful of over-the-counter and professionally prescribed prescriptions. Adhere to dosing directions and counsel a medical care supplier in the event that you have concerns.

7. **Avoid Toxins**: Limit openness to ecological poisons and synthetic substances that can hurt your liver.

8. **Regular Check-ups**: Visit your medical care supplier for normal check-ups and screenings,

particularly assuming you have risk factors for liver infection.

So the liver is an imperative organ with a large number of capabilities in the body. Liver illness can have serious results, however it is preventable and reasonable through way of life decisions and early location. By embracing a solid way of life, remaining informed about risk factors, and looking for clinical counsel when required, you can safeguard your liver and by and large prosperity. Liver illness ought not be messed with, and everybody can find straightforward ways to guarantee the strength of this fundamental organ.

CHAPTER 2

2.1 Maintain fatty liver disease diet to achieve optimum health.

A greasy liver illness diet assumes a pivotal part in dealing with this condition and advancing ideal wellbeing. Greasy liver illness, portrayed by the gathering of abundant fat in the liver, can be of two sorts. non-alcoholic greasy liver sickness (NAFLD) and alcoholic greasy liver illness (AFLD). While dietary suggestions can differ somewhat between these two kinds, there are common rules that can assist people with accomplishing ideal wellbeing.

2.2 Food sources to Eat

A. **Leafy foods**: Integrate different vivid products of the soil into your eating regimen. They are plentiful in cancer prevention agents, nutrients, and fiber that assist with diminishing aggravation and backing liver wellbeing. Hold back nothing 5 servings per day.

B. **Entire Grains**: Pick entire grains like earthy colored rice, quinoa, and entire wheat bread. These give complex starches, fiber, and supplements that balance out glucose levels and advance satiety.

C. **Lean Proteins**: Decide on lean protein sources like skinless poultry, fish, tofu, and vegetables. Protein is fundamental for liver fix and capability without the additional immersed fats tracked down in red meat.

D. **Sound Fats**: Incorporate wellsprings of solid fats like avocados, nuts, seeds, and olive oil. These facts are valuable for generally wellbeing and can decrease aggravation in the liver.

E. **Greasy Fish**: Greasy fish like salmon, mackerel, and sardines are wealthy in omega-3 unsaturated fats, which have calming properties and back liver wellbeing.

F. **Dairy**: Pick low-fat or sans fat dairy items to diminish the admission of immersed fats. Dairy gives fundamental supplements like calcium, which is significant for bone wellbeing.

2.3   Food sources to Avoid

A. **Sweet Foods**: Limit your utilization of sweet food sources and beverages, including pop, treats, and pastries. Unreasonable sugar admission can prompt insulin opposition and deteriorate NAFLD.

B. **Handled Foods**: Exceptionally handled food varieties are frequently stacked with unfortunate fats, sugars, and added substances. These can fuel liver aggravation and add to weight gain.

C. **Soaked Fats**: Breaking point food varieties high in immersed fats, like red meat, spread, and full-fat dairy items. Soaked fats can add to liver fat aggregation.

D. **Trans Fats**: Stay away from trans fats tracked down in many quick food sources, bundled snacks, and seared food varieties. Trans fats are known to be destructive to the liver and generally wellbeing.

E. **Unreasonable Alcohol**: For people with NAFLD, liquor utilization ought to be negligible or stayed away from altogether. For those with AFLD, halting drinking liquor altogether is basic.

2.4   Segment Control and Calorie Intake

Controlling piece estimates and overseeing calorie admission is fundamental for accomplishing and keeping a solid weight. Abundant calories, even from good food sources, can add to fat collection in the liver. Talk with a medical services proficient or dietitian to decide the suitable everyday calorie consumption for your particular necessities.

Hydration

Remaining very much hydrated is fundamental for liver capability. Water helps flush poisons from the body and supports by and large wellbeing. Limit the utilization of sweet drinks and select water or home grown teas.

Ordinary Exercise

Consolidating a solid eating regimen with ordinary actual work is crucial for overseeing greasy liver sickness. Practice further develops insulin awareness, helps with weight reduction, and supports generally speaking liver wellbeing.

Clinical Supervision

It's essential to work intimately with a medical care supplier or an enrolled dietitian to make a customized diet plan that tends to your particular requirements and the sort and seriousness of your greasy liver infection.

So in accomplishing ideal wellbeing with a greasy liver sickness diet includes a reasonable and nutritious methodology. Focusing on entire, natural food sources, keeping away from destructive fixings, keeping up with segment control, and integrating normal activity into your routine can go far in overseeing and working on the condition. Recall that dietary changes ought to be made in conference with medical care experts to guarantee the most ideal results for your liver wellbeing.

2.5   Benefits of following a fatty liver disease diet

1. **Weight Management**: Keeping a solid weight is pivotal for overseeing greasy liver sickness. The eating regimen can assist you with lessening overabundance of muscle versus fat, which is an essential driver of the condition.

2. **Reduced Fat Accumulation**: The eating routine ordinarily restricts the admission of soaked and trans fats, which can forestall further fat development in the liver.

3. **Improved Insulin Sensitivity**: A greasy liver eating regimen frequently underscores complex starches, fiber, and lean proteins, which can assist with further developing insulin responsiveness and better control glucose levels.

4. **Liver Health**: It advances the utilization of food sources that help liver wellbeing, like organic products, vegetables, and food sources wealthy in cell reinforcements and mitigating compounds.

5. **Lowering Blood Lipids**: A greasy liver eating routine can assist with decreasing raised blood lipid levels, including fatty oils and LDL cholesterol.

6. **Reduced Inflammation**: The eating routine can assist with diminishing irritation in the body, which is significant for overseeing and forestalling the movement of liver illness.

7. **Balanced Nutrition**: It empowers an even admission of supplements, guaranteeing that the body gets fundamental and minerals.

8. **Improved General Health**: By advancing a heart-sound, adjusted diet, following a greasy liver sickness diet can help your general wellbeing, diminishing the gamble of different circumstances like coronary illness and diabetes.

Keep in mind, it's fundamental to talk with a medical care proficient or enrolled dietitian to foster a customized diet plan custom-made to your particular requirements and ailment.

CHAPTER 3

3.1 Complications of fatty liver disease, if the right diet isn't adopted.

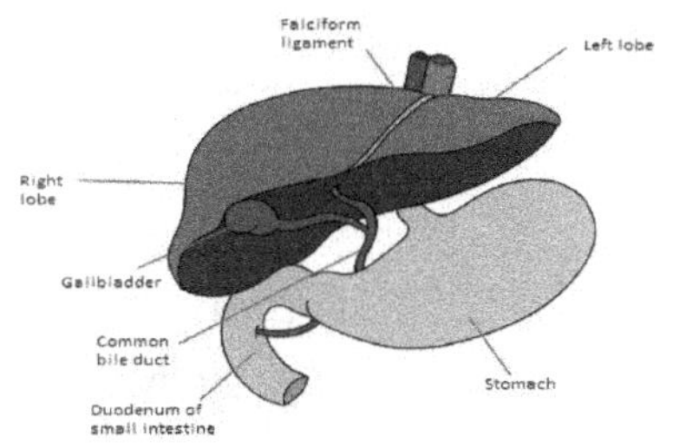

In the event that a legitimate eating routine and way of life changes are not taken on to oversee greasy liver illness (non-alcoholic greasy liver sickness - NAFLD), it can prompt different confusions.

1. **NASH (Non-Alcoholic Steatohepatitis):** Movement of NAFLD to NASH, a more extreme structure, which can cause liver irritation and scarring (fibrosis).

2. **Liver Fibrosis**: Proceeded with aggravation might prompt fibrosis, where liver tissue becomes scarred. This can decrease liver capability over the long run.

3. **Cirrhosis**: In cutting edge stages, broad liver fibrosis can form into cirrhosis, a condition where the liver turns out to be seriously scarred, disabling its capability.

4. **Liver Failure**: Cirrhosis can advance to liver disappointment, where the liver can never again carry out its fundamental roles, possibly requiring a liver transfer.

5. **Hepatocellular Carcinoma (Liver Cancer**): People with cutting edge greasy liver infection have a higher gamble of creating liver malignant growth.

6.**Cardiovascular Complications**: Greasy liver sickness is frequently connected with metabolic condition, which expands the gamble of coronary illness, hypertension, and diabetes.

7. **Kidney Disease**: There is a connection among NAFLD and kidney illness, and the presence of greasy liver can fuel kidney issues.

8. **Sleep Apnea**: Greasy liver infection can add to rest apnea, which further deteriorates generally wellbeing.

9. **Osteoporosis**: Individuals with NAFLD might be at a higher gamble of bone breaks because of an absence of vitamin D ingestion.

10. **Psychological Impact**: The pressure and stress related to liver sickness can prompt close to home and psychological well-being issues.

It's vital to embrace a sound way of life and dietary changes to oversee and possibly invert greasy liver sickness. Ordinary clinical observing and conference with medical care experts are critical to actually forestall and deal with these inconveniences.

CHAPTER 4

BREAKFAST RECIPES
1. Avocado and Spinach Breakfast Bowl

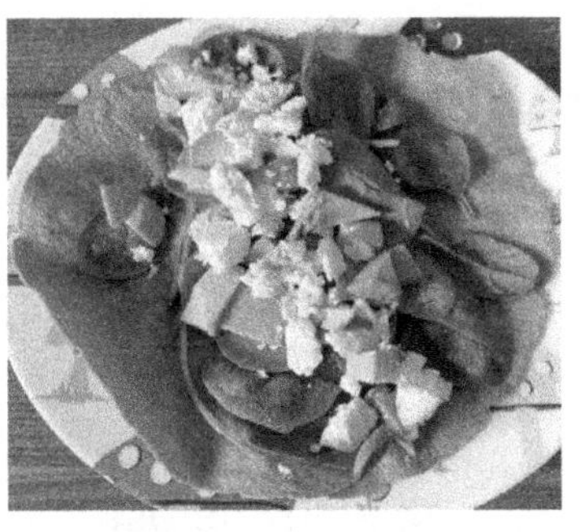

Nutritional Value (approx.)

- Calories. 300
- Protein. 10g
- Carbohydrates. 15g
- Fiber. 7g
- **Prep. Time:** 15 min

Ingredients:

- 1 ripe avocado
- 2 cups fresh spinach leaves
- 1 poached egg
- 1 teaspoon olive oil
- Salt and pepper to taste

Instructions:

1. Mash the avocado and season with salt and pepper.
2. Sauté spinach in olive oil until wilted.
3. Top spinach with mashed avocado and a poached egg.
4. Serve immediately.

2. Oatmeal with Berries and Almonds

ingredients:

- 1/2 cup rolled oats
- 1 cup unsweetened almond milk
- 1/4 cup fresh berries (blueberries, strawberries)
- 1 tablespoon sliced almonds
- 1 teaspoon honey (optional)

Instructions:

1. Cook oats in almond milk until creamy.
2. Top with berries, almonds, and a drizzle of honey if desired.

Nutritional Value (approx.).
- Calories. 250
- Protein. 6g
- Carbohydrates. 35g
- Fiber. 8g
- **Prep. Time:** 10 minutes

3. Greek Yogurt Parfait

Ingredients:

- 1 cup Greek yogurt
- 1/2 cup granola (low sugar)
- 1/4 cup fresh mixed berries
- 1 tablespoon honey

Instructions:

1. Layer Greek yogurt, granola, and berries in a glass.
2. Drizzle with honey.

Nutritional Value (approx.)
- Calories. 350
- Protein. 15g
- Carbohydrates. 40g
- Fiber. 5g

Prep. Time: 5 minutes

4. Spinach and Mushroom Omelette

Ingredients:
- 2 large eggs
- 1 cup fresh spinach, chopped
- 1/4 cup sliced mushrooms
- 1/4 cup diced onions
- 1/4 cup low-fat cheese (optional)
- 1 teaspoon olive oil
- Salt and pepper to taste

Instructions:

1. In a pan, sauté mushrooms and onions in olive oil until tender.

2. Whisk eggs, season with salt and pepper, and pour over sautéed vegetables.

3. Cook until the omelet is set, and add cheese if desired.

Nutritional Value (approx.)
- Calories. 300
- Protein. 20g
- Carbohydrates. 7g
- Fiber. 2g

Prep. Time: 15 minutes

5. Quinoa and Fruit Breakfast Bowl

Ingredients:

- 1/2 cup cooked quinoa
- 1/2 cup low-fat yogurt
- 1/4 cup fresh mixed fruit (e.g., mango, pineapple, kiwi)
- 1 tablespoon chopped nuts (almonds or walnuts)
- 1 teaspoon honey (optional)

Instructions:

1. Layer cooked quinoa with yogurt and mixed fruit.
2. Top with nuts and drizzle with honey if desired.

Nutritional Value (approx.)
- Calories. 300
- Protein. 10g
- Carbohydrates. 45g
- Fiber. 6g
Prep. Time: 10 minutes

6. Sweet Potato Hash

Ingredients:

- 1 medium sweet potato, diced
- 1/4 cup diced bell peppers
- 1/4 cup diced onions
- 1 tablespoon olive oil
- 1/4 teaspoon paprika
- Salt and pepper to taste

Instructions:

1. Heat olive oil in a skillet and sauté sweet potatoes, bell peppers, and onions until tender.

2. Season with paprika, salt, and pepper.

Nutritional Value (approx.)

- Calories. 250
- Protein. 3g
- Carbohydrates. 40g
- Fiber. 6g
- **Prep. Time:** 20 minutes

7. Chia Seed Pudding

Ingredients:

- 3 tablespoons chia seeds
- 1 cup unsweetened almond milk
- 1/2 teaspoon vanilla extract
- 1/4 cup fresh berries
- 1 teaspoon honey (optional)

Instructions:

1. Mix chia seeds, almond milk, and vanilla extract in a bowl. Let it sit for a few hours or overnight to thicken.
2. Top with fresh berries and a drizzle of honey.

Nutritional Value (approx.)
- Calories. 200
- Protein. 6g
- Carbohydrates. 20g
- Fiber. 14g

Prep. Time: 5 minutes (plus chilling time)

8. Banana and Almond Butter Toast

Ingredients:

- 1 slice of whole-grain bread
- 1 ripe banana, sliced
- 1 tablespoon almond butter
- Cinnamon (optional)

Instructions:

1. Toast the whole-grain bread.
2. Spread almond butter on the toast and top with banana slices.
3. Sprinkle with a dash of cinnamon if desired.

Nutritional Value (approx.)
- Calories. 250
- Protein. 7g
- Carbohydrates. 40g
- Fiber. 7g
Prep. Time: 5 minutes

9. Cottage Cheese and Berries Bowl

Ingredients:
- 1/2 cup low-fat cottage cheese
- 1/2 cup mixed berries (blueberries, raspberries)
- 1 tablespoon chopped nuts (e.g., almonds, walnuts)
- 1 teaspoon honey (optional)

Instructions:
1. In a bowl, layer cottage cheese with mixed berries.
2. Top with chopped nuts and drizzle with honey if desired.

Nutritional Value (approx.)
- Calories. 220
- Protein. 15g
- Carbohydrates. 20g
- Fiber. 4g

Prep. Time: 5 minutes

10. Veggie and Egg Breakfast Wrap

Ingredients:

- 1 whole-grain tortilla
- 2 large eggs
- 1/4 cup diced bell peppers
- 1/4 cup diced onions
- 1/4 cup diced tomatoes
- 1 teaspoon olive oil
- Salt and pepper to taste

Instructions:

1. Sauté vegetables in olive oil until tender.
2. Scramble eggs and add to the sautéed vegetables.
3. Spoon the egg and veggie mixture onto the whole-grain tortilla, wrap, and enjoy.

Nutritional Value (approx.)
- Calories. 300
- Protein. 15g
- Carbohydrates. 25g
- Fiber. 6g

Prep. Time: 15 minutes

11. Salmon and Cream Cheese Toast

Ingredients:

- 1 slice of whole-grain bread
- 2 ounces smoked salmon
- 2 tablespoons low-fat cream cheese
- Fresh dill (optional)

Instructions:

1. Toast the whole-grain bread.
2. Spread cream cheese on the toast.
3. Top with smoked salmon and a garnish of fresh dill if desired.

Nutritional Value (approx.)
- Calories. 300
- Protein. 20g
- Carbohydrates. 20g
- Fiber. 4g

Prep. Time: 5 minutes

12. Berry and Spinach Smoothie

Ingredients:

- 1 cup fresh spinach

- 1/2 cup mixed berries (strawberries, blueberries)
- 1/2 cup low-fat yogurt
- 1/2 cup water or unsweetened almond milk
- 1 tablespoon chia seeds

Instructions:

1. Blend spinach, berries, yogurt, and liquid until smooth.
2. Stir in chia seeds and let it sit for a few minutes to thicken.

Nutritional Value (approx.)
- Calories. 250
- Protein. 8g
- Carbohydrates. 30g
- Fiber. 10g

Prep. Time: 5 minutes

CHAPTER 5

LUNCH RECIPES

13. Grilled Chicken and Vegetable Salad

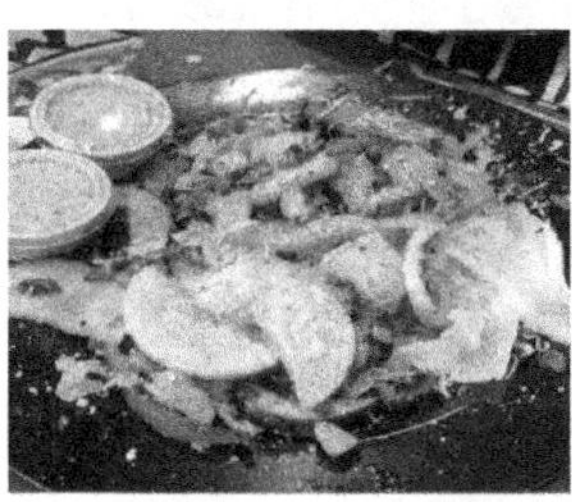

Nutritional Value (approx.)
- Calories. 300
- Protein. 30g
- Carbohydrates. 12g
- Fiber. 4g

Prep. Time: 20 minutes

Ingredients:

- 4 oz (120g) boneless, skinless chicken breast
- 2 cups mixed greens (lettuce, spinach)
- 1/2 cup cherry tomatoes
- 1/4 cup cucumber slices
- 1/4 cup bell pepper strips
- 1 tablespoon balsamic vinaigrette (low-fat)

Instructions:

1. Grill the chicken breast until fully cooked.

2. Slice the grilled chicken and arrange it over the mixed greens.

3. Add cherry tomatoes, cucumber, and bell peppers.

4. Drizzle with balsamic vinaigrette.

14. Quinoa and Black Bean Salad

Ingredients:

- 1/2 cup cooked quinoa
- 1/2 cup black beans (canned and rinsed)
- 1/4 cup corn kernels
- 1/4 cup diced red onion
- 1/4 cup chopped cilantro
- 2 tablespoons lime juice

Instructions:

1. Combine quinoa, black beans, corn, red onion, and cilantro in a bowl.
2. Drizzle with lime juice and toss to mix.

Nutritional Value (approx.)
- Calories. 320
- Protein. 11g
- Carbohydrates. 60g
- Fiber. 10g

Prep. Time: 15 minutes

15. Tuna and White Bean Salad

Ingredients:

- 4 oz (120g) canned tuna in water, drained
- 1/2 cup canned white beans (cannellini), drained and rinsed
- 1/4 cup diced red onion
- 1/4 cup diced celery
- 1 tablespoon lemon juice
- 1 tablespoon olive oil

- Instructions:

1. In a bowl, combine tuna, white beans, red onion, and celery.
2. Drizzle with lemon juice and olive oil, and gently mix.

Nutritional Value (approx.)
- Calories. 280
- Protein. 25g
- Carbohydrates. 18g
- Fiber. 6g

Prep. Time: 10 minutes

16. Lentil and Vegetable Soup

Ingredients:

- 1/2 cup dried green or brown lentils
- 2 cups low-sodium vegetable broth
- 1/2 cup diced carrots
- 1/2 cup diced celery
- 1/2 cup diced zucchini
- 1/2 cup diced tomatoes
- 1 teaspoon olive oil
- Seasonings (thyme, bay leaf, salt, and pepper to taste)

Instructions:

1. In a pot, sauté carrots, celery, and zucchini in olive oil.

2. Add lentils, diced tomatoes, vegetable broth, and seasonings.

3. Simmer until lentils and vegetables are tender.

Nutritional Value (approx.)
- Calories. 250
- Protein. 12g
- Carbohydrates. 40g
- Fiber. 10g

Prep. Time: 30 minutes

17. Baked Salmon with Roasted Vegetables

Ingredients:
- 4 oz (120g) salmon filet

- 1 cup mixed roasted vegetables (zucchini, bell peppers, cherry tomatoes)
- 1 teaspoon olive oil
- Lemon wedges
- Seasonings (rosemary, garlic, salt, and pepper to taste)

Instructions:

1. Season salmon with rosemary, garlic, salt, and pepper.
2. Bake salmon in the oven.
3. Toss the mixed roasted vegetables in olive oil and roast until tender.
4. Serve with lemon wedges.

Nutritional Value (approx.)

- Calories. 350
- Protein. 25g
- Carbohydrates. 15g
- Fiber. 4g

Prep. Time: 30 minutes

18. Chickpea and Cucumber Salad

Ingredients:

- 1 cup canned chickpeas, drained and rinsed
- 1/2 cup diced cucumber

- 1/4 cup diced red onion
- 1/4 cup chopped parsley
- 2 tablespoons lemon juice
- 1 tablespoon olive oil

Instructions:

1. Combine chickpeas, cucumber, red onion, and parsley in a bowl.

2. Drizzle with lemon juice and olive oil, and toss to mix.

Nutritional Value (approx.)

- Calories. 280
- Protein. 10g
- Carbohydrates. 40g
- Fiber. 10g

Prep. Time: 10 minutes

19. Turkey and Avocado Wrap

Ingredients:
- 2 slices of whole-grain tortilla
- 3 oz (85g) sliced turkey breast
- 1/4 avocado, sliced
- 1/2 cup mixed greens
- Mustard or low-fat mayonnaise (optional)

Instructions:
1. Lay out the tortilla and add turkey, avocado, and mixed greens.
2. Optionally, spread with mustard or low-fat mayo.
3. Roll up and serve.

Nutritional Value (approx.)
- Calories. 300
- Protein. 20g
- Carbohydrates. 30g
- Fiber. 8g

Prep. Time: 10 minutes

20. Spinach and Feta Stuffed Chicken Breast

Ingredients:

- 4 oz (120g) chicken breast
- 1 cup fresh spinach
- 2 tablespoons crumbled feta cheese
- 1 teaspoon olive oil
- Seasonings (garlic, oregano, salt, and pepper to taste)

Instructions:

1. Butterfly the chicken breast and season it.
2. Sauté fresh spinach in olive oil.
3. Stuff the chicken breast with sautéed spinach and feta.
4. Bake until the chicken is cooked through.

- **Nutritional Value (approx.)**
  - Calories. 280
  - Protein. 30g
  - Carbohydrates. 2g
  - Fiber. 1g

Prep. Time: 35 minutes

21. Quinoa and Roasted Vegetable Bowl

Ingredients:
- 1/2 cup cooked quinoa
- 1 cup roasted mixed vegetables (bell peppers, zucchini, eggplant)
- 1/4 cup crumbled goat cheese
- 2 tablespoons balsamic vinaigrette (low-fat)

Instructions:
1. Combine cooked quinoa and roasted vegetables in a bowl.
2. Top with crumbled goat cheese and drizzle with balsamic vinaigrette.

Nutritional Value (approx.)
- Calories. 320
- Protein. 10g
- Carbohydrates. 40g
- Fiber. 8g

Prep. Time: 25 minutes

22. Shrimp and Broccoli Stir-Fry

Ingredients:
- 4 oz (120g) shrimp, peeled and deveined
- 1 cup broccoli florets
- 1/4 cup sliced red bell pepper
- 1/4 cup sliced carrots
- 2 tablespoons low-sodium soy sauce
- 1 tablespoon olive oil

Instructions:
1. In a pan, sauté shrimp, broccoli, red bell pepper, and carrots in olive oil.
2. Add low-sodium soy sauce and stir-fry until cooked.

Nutritional Value (approx.)
- Calories. 280
- Protein. 25g
- Carbohydrates. 10g
- Fiber. 4g

Prep. Time: 20 minutes.

CHAPTER 6

DINNER RECIPES

23. Baked Salmon with Asparagus

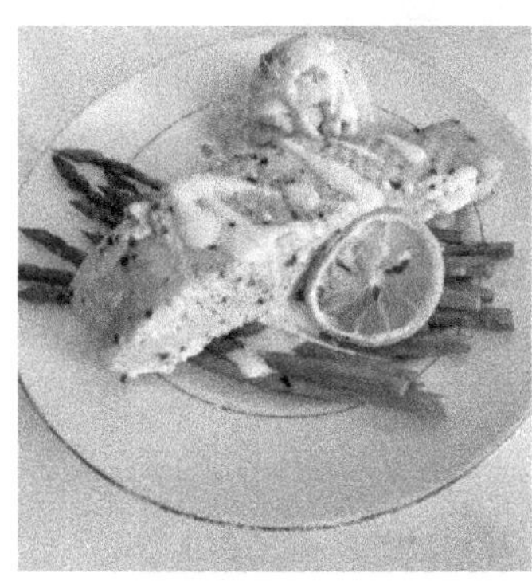

Nutritional Value (approx.)
- Calories. 350
- Protein. 30g
- Carbohydrates. 6g
- Fiber. 3g

Prep. Time: 25 minutes

Ingredients:

- 6 oz (170g) salmon filet
- 1 cup asparagus spears
- 1 tablespoon olive oil
- Lemon slices
- Seasonings (garlic, dill, salt, and pepper to taste)

Instructions:

1. Preheat the oven to 375°F (190°C).
2. Place salmon and asparagus on a baking sheet.
3. Drizzle with olive oil, season with garlic, dill, salt, and pepper.
4. Bake until the salmon flakes easily and asparagus is tender.
5. Serve with lemon slices.

24. Quinoa and Black Bean Stuffed Peppers

Ingredients:

- 2 large bell peppers
- 1/2 cup cooked quinoa
- 1/2 cup canned black beans, drained and rinsed
- 1/4 cup diced tomatoes
- 1/4 cup diced onions
- 2 tablespoons low-sodium salsa

Instructions:

1. Cut the tops off the peppers and remove seeds.
2. In a bowl, mix quinoa, black beans, diced tomatoes, onions, and salsa.
3. Stuff the peppers with the quinoa mixture.
4. Bake until peppers are tender.

Nutritional Value (approx.)

- Calories. 320
- Protein. 12g
- Carbohydrates. 60g
- Fiber. 12g

Prep. Time: 40 minutes

25. Grilled Chicken with Roasted Vegetables

Ingredients:

- 6 oz (170g) boneless, skinless chicken breast

- 1 cup mixed roasted vegetables (zucchini, bell peppers, eggplant)
- 1 tablespoon olive oil
- Seasonings (rosemary, garlic, salt, and pepper to taste)

Instructions:

1. Season chicken with rosemary, garlic, salt, and pepper.
2. Grill the chicken until fully cooked.
3. Toss the mixed roasted vegetables in olive oil and roast until tender.

Nutritional Value (approx.)
- Calories. 350
- Protein. 35g
- Carbohydrates. 20g
- Fiber. 8g

Prep. Time: 30 minutes

26. Turkey and Vegetable Stir-Fry

Ingredients:

- 6 oz (170g) ground turkey
- 1 cup mixed stir-fry vegetables (broccoli, bell peppers, snap peas)

- 1 tablespoon low-sodium soy sauce
- 1 tablespoon olive oil
- Ginger and garlic (for flavor)

Instructions:

1. In a pan, sauté ground turkey with ginger and garlic until browned.
2. Add mixed stir-fry vegetables and stir-fry until tender.
3. Drizzle with low-sodium soy sauce.

Nutritional Value (approx.)
- Calories. 320
- Protein. 30g
- Carbohydrates. 10g
- Fiber. 4g

Prep. Time: 20 minutes

27. Lentil and Spinach Curry

Ingredients:

- 1/2 cup dried green or brown lentils
- 2 cups fresh spinach
- 1/2 cup diced tomatoes
- 1/4 cup diced onions
- 2 tablespoons low-sodium curry paste

- Seasonings (cumin, coriander, salt, and pepper to taste)

Instructions:

1. Cook lentils in water until tender.
2. In a pan, sauté onions and spices.
3. Add diced tomatoes and cook until they soften.
4. Stir in cooked lentils and fresh spinach.
5. Mix in low-sodium curry paste.

Nutritional Value (approx.)
- Calories. 320
- Protein. 15g
- Carbohydrates. 50g
- Fiber. 15g

Prep. Time: 30 minutes

28. Shrimp and Broccoli Quinoa Bowl

Ingredients:

- 4 oz (120g) shrimp, peeled and deveined
- 1 cup steamed broccoli florets
- 1/2 cup cooked quinoa
- 1 tablespoon low-sodium teriyaki sauce
- Sesame seeds for garnish

- Instructions:

1. Sauté shrimp in a pan until cooked.
2. In a bowl, combine cooked quinoa, steamed broccoli, and shrimp.
3. Drizzle with low-sodium teriyaki sauce.
4. Garnish with sesame seeds.

- **Nutritional Value (approx.)**
  - Calories. 350
  - Protein. 25g
  - Carbohydrates. 40g
  - Fiber. 5g
Prep. Time: 25 minutes

29. Tofu and Vegetable Stir-Fry

Ingredients:

- 6 oz (170g) firm tofu, cubed
- 1 cup mixed stir-fry vegetables (snow peas, bell peppers, carrots)
- 1 tablespoon low-sodium stir-fry sauce
- 1 tablespoon sesame oil
- Ginger and garlic (for flavor)

Instructions:

1. In a wok, stir-fry tofu with ginger and garlic until golden.
2. Add mixed vegetables and stir-fry until tender.
3. Drizzle with low-sodium stir-fry sauce and sesame oil.

Nutritional Value (approx.)
- Calories. 330
- Protein. 15g
- Carbohydrates. 20g
- Fiber. 5g
Prep. Time: 30 minutes

30. Lemon Herb Baked Chicken

Ingredients:

- 6 oz (170g) chicken breast
- 1 lemon, sliced
- 1 tablespoon olive oil
- Fresh herbs (such as rosemary, thyme)
- Salt and pepper to taste

Instructions:

1. Preheat the oven to 375°F (190°C).
2. Place the chicken breast in a baking dish.

3. Drizzle with olive oil, season with salt, pepper, and herbs.

4. Lay lemon slices on top.

5. Bake until the chicken is cooked through.

Nutritional Value (approx.)
- Calories. 300
- Protein. 35g
- Carbohydrates. 2g
- Fiber. 1g

Prep. Time: 30 minutes

31. Baked Cod with Salsa

Ingredients:

- 6 oz (170g) cod filet
- 1/2 cup diced tomatoes
- 1/4 cup diced onions
- 1/4 cup diced bell peppers
- 1/4 cup chopped cilantro
- 1 tablespoon olive oil
- Lime juice, to taste

- Instructions:

1. Preheat the oven to 375°F (190°C).
2. Place cod in a baking dish.
3. Mix tomatoes, onions, bell peppers, and cilantro.
4. Drizzle with olive oil and lime juice.
5. Spoon the salsa over the cod.
6. Bake until the cod is cooked through.

- Nutritional Value (approx.)
- Calories. 280
- Protein. 30g
- Carbohydrates. 10g
- Fiber. 3g

Prep. Time: 25 minutes

32. Eggplant and Lentil Stew

Ingredients:

- 1/2 cup dried brown lentils
- 1 medium eggplant, diced
- 1/4 cup diced tomatoes
- 1/4 cup diced onions
- 2 cloves garlic, minced
- 1 tablespoon olive oil
- Seasonings (cumin, coriander, salt, and pepper to taste)

Instructions:

1. Cook lentils until tender.
2. In a pot, sauté onions and garlic in olive oil.
3. Add eggplant and cook until softened.
4. Stir in diced tomatoes, cooked lentils, and seasonings.
5. Simmer until the stew is heated through.

Nutritional Value (approx.)
- Calories. 320
- Protein. 13g
- Carbohydrates. 55g
- Fiber. 15g
Prep. Time: 35 minutes

CHAPTER 7

SNACKS RECIPES
33. Greek Yogurt and Berry Parfait

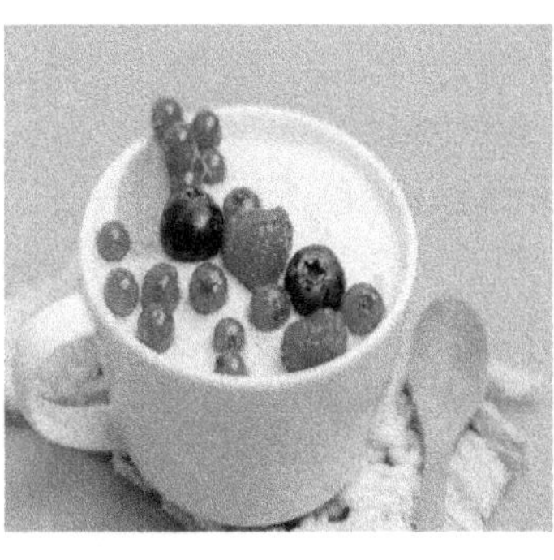

Nutritional Value (approx.)
- Calories. 200
- Protein. 15g
- Carbohydrates. 30g
- Fiber. 5g

Prep. Time: 5 minutes

Ingredients:

- 1 cup low-fat Greek yogurt
- 1/2 cup mixed berries (blueberries, strawberries)
- 1 tablespoon honey (optional)

Instructions:

1. In a glass, layer Greek yogurt and mixed berries.
2. Drizzle with honey if desired.

34. Apple Slices with Almond Butter

Ingredients:
- 1 medium apple, sliced
- 2 tablespoons almond butter

Instructions:
1. Slice the apple into thin wedges.
2. Dip apple slices in almond butter.

Nutritional Value (approx.)
- Calories. 250
- Protein. 6g
- Carbohydrates. 25g
- Fiber. 6g

Prep. Time: 5 minutes

35. Cucumber and Hummus

Ingredients:
- 1 medium cucumber, sliced
- 1/4 cup hummus

Instructions:
1. Slice the cucumber into rounds or sticks.
2. Dip cucumber slices in hummus.

Nutritional Value (approx.).
- Calories. 150
- Protein. 6g
- Carbohydrates. 15g
- Fiber. 5g

Prep. Time: 5 minutes

36. Hard-Boiled Eggs

Ingredients:
- 2 hard-boiled eggs

Instructions:
1. Boil the eggs until they are hard-boiled.
2. Peel and slice the eggs.

Nutritional Value (approx. per egg).

- Calories. 70
- Protein. 6g
- Carbohydrates. 0g
- Fiber. 0g
Prep. Time: 15 minutes (includes boiling)

40. Mixed Nuts

Ingredients:

- 1/4 cup mixed unsalted nuts (almonds, walnuts, cashews)

- Instructions:
1. Measure the mixed nuts and enjoy as a snack.

Nutritional Value (approx.)
- Calories. 200
- Protein. 5g
- Carbohydrates. 7g
- Fiber. 3g
Prep. Time: Instant

42. Carrot and Hummus

Ingredients:
- 1 medium carrot, sliced into sticks
- 1/4 cup hummus

Instructions:

1. Slice the carrot into sticks or rounds.
2. Dip carrot sticks into hummus.

Nutritional Value (approx.).
- Calories. 120
- Protein. 3g
- Carbohydrates. 15g
- Fiber. 4g

Prep. Time: 5 minutes

43. Cottage Cheese with Pineapple

Ingredients:
- 1/2 cup low-fat cottage cheese
- 1/4 cup diced fresh pineapple

Instructions:

1. In a bowl, combine cottage cheese and diced pineapple.
2. Mix well and enjoy.

Nutritional Value (approx.)
- Calories. 150
- Protein. 15g
- Carbohydrates. 15g
- Fiber. 1g

Prep. Time: 5 minutes

44. Whole Wheat Toast with Avocado

Ingredients:
- 1 slice of whole wheat toast
- 1/4 ripe avocado, mashed
- Red pepper flakes (optional)

Instructions:
1. Toast the whole wheat bread.
2. Spread mashed avocado on the toast.
3. Add a dash of red pepper flakes if desired.

Nutritional Value (approx.)
- Calories. 150
- Protein. 3g
- Carbohydrates. 15g
- Fiber. 4g

Prep. Time: 5 minutes

45. Berry and Spinach Smoothie

Ingredients:
- 1 cup fresh spinach
- 1/2 cup mixed berries (strawberries, blueberries)
- 1/2 cup low-fat yogurt
- 1/2 cup water or unsweetened almond milk
- 1 tablespoon chia seeds

Instructions:

1. Blend spinach, berries, yogurt, and liquid until smooth.

2. Stir in chia seeds and let it sit for a few minutes to thicken.

Nutritional Value (approx.)
- Calories. 250
- Protein. 8g
- Carbohydrates. 30g
- Fiber. 10g

Prep. Time: 5 minutes (plus chilling time)

46. Sliced Bell Peppers with Guacamole

Ingredients:
- 1 medium bell pepper, sliced
- 1/4 cup homemade guacamole (avocado, lime juice, garlic, salt)

Instructions:
1. Slice the bell pepper into strips.
2. Dip pepper strips in homemade guacamole.

Nutritional Value (approx.)
- Calories. 120
- Protein. 2g
- Carbohydrates. 10g
- Fiber. 4g

Prep. Time: 10 minutes

CHAPTER 8

POULTRY AND MEAT

47.Grilled Chicken Breast with Lemon and Herbs

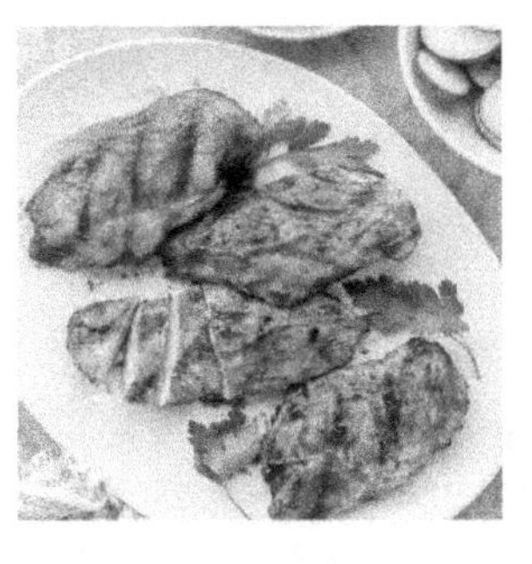

Nutritional value (approx. per serving):
Calories. 200
Protein. 30g
Carbohydrates. 2g
Fiber. 0g
Preparation Time: 40 minutes (includes marinating and grilling)

Ingredients:

- 2 boneless, skinless chicken breasts (6 oz each)
- 1 lemon, juiced
- 2 cloves garlic, minced
- 1 teaspoon fresh thyme
- Salt and pepper to taste

Instructions:

1. In a bowl, mix lemon juice, minced garlic, thyme, salt, and pepper.

2. Marinate chicken breasts in the mixture for 30 minutes.

3. Grill the chicken until fully cooked.

48. Turkey and Vegetable Skewers

Ingredients:

- 8 oz (225g) lean ground turkey
- 1/2 cup bell pepper, cut into chunks
- 1/2 cup zucchini, cut into chunks
- 1/4 cup red onion, cut into chunks
- 1 tablespoon olive oil
- Seasonings (oregano, paprika, salt, and pepper to taste)

Instructions:

1. In a bowl, mix ground turkey with seasonings.
2. Form turkey into small meatballs.
3. Thread turkey meatballs and vegetables onto skewers.
4. Brush with olive oil and grill until turkey is cooked through.

Nutritional Value. (approx. per serving).
- Calories. 250
- Protein. 25g
- Carbohydrates. 6g
- Fiber. 2g

Prep. Time: 30 minutes (includes grilling)

49. Baked Salmon with Dill and Mustard Sauce

Ingredients:
- 2 salmon filets (6 oz each)
- 2 tablespoons Dijon mustard
- 1 tablespoon fresh dill

- • 1 tablespoon olive oil
- • Lemon wedges

Instructions:
1. Preheat the oven to 375°F (190°C).
2. In a bowl, mix Dijon mustard, fresh dill, and olive oil.
3. Coat salmon with the mustard mixture.
4. Bake until the salmon flakes easily.
5. Serve with lemon wedges.

Nutritional value (approx. per serving):
- Calories. 300
- Protein. 35g
- Carbohydrates. 2g
- Fiber. 0g

Prep. Time: 20 minutes (including baking)

50. Lean Beef Stir-Fry

Ingredients:
- 6 oz (170g) lean beef strips
- 1 cup mixed stir-fry vegetables (broccoli, bell peppers, snap peas)
- 1 tablespoon low-sodium soy sauce
- 1 tablespoon olive oil
- Ginger and garlic (for flavor)

Instructions:
1. In a wok, stir-fry beef with ginger and garlic until browned.
2. Add mixed vegetables and stir-fry until tender.
3. Drizzle with low-sodium soy sauce.

Nutritional value (approx. per serving):
- Calories. 280
- Protein. 30g
- Carbohydrates. 10g
- Fiber. 3g

Prep. Time: 20 minutes

51. Herbed Pork Chops with Roasted Vegetables

Ingredients:

- 2 boneless pork chops (6 oz each)
- 1 cup mixed roasted vegetables (zucchini, bell peppers, cherry tomatoes)
- 1 tablespoon olive oil
- Seasonings (rosemary, garlic, salt, and pepper to taste)

Instructions:

1. Season pork chops with rosemary, garlic, salt, and pepper.
2. Grill pork chops until fully cooked.
3. Toss the mixed roasted vegetables in olive oil and roast until tender.

Nutritional value (approx. per serving):

- Calories. 320
- Protein. 30g
- Carbohydrates. 15g
- Fiber. 4g

Prep. Time: 30 minutes

CHAPTER 9

52. Baked Salmon with Lemon and Dill

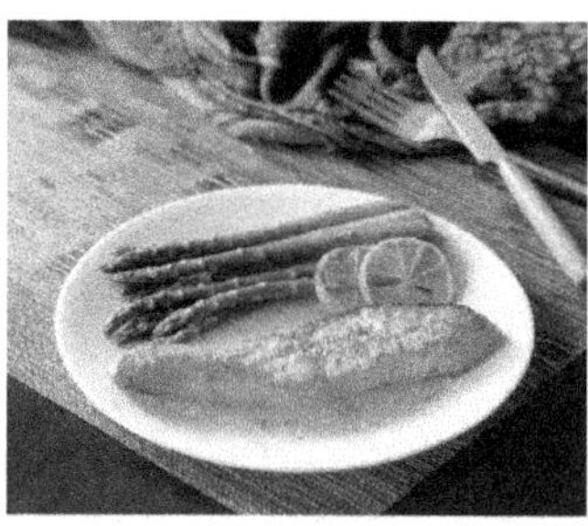

Nutritional value (approx. per serving):
Calories. 300
Protein. 30g
Carbohydrates. 2g
Fiber. 0g
Prep. Time: 20 minutes

Ingredients:

- 2 salmon filets (6 oz each)
- 1 lemon, juiced and zested
- 1 tablespoon fresh dill
- Salt and pepper to taste
- Olive oil for drizzling

Instructions:

1. Preheat the oven to 375°F (190°C).
2. Season salmon filets with lemon zest, dill, salt, and pepper.
3. Drizzle with lemon juice and olive oil.
4. Bake until salmon is cooked through.

53. Grilled Shrimp and Vegetable Skewers

Ingredients:

- 8 oz (225g) large shrimp, peeled and deveined
- 1/2 cup bell peppers, cut into chunks
- 1/2 cup zucchini, cut into chunks
- 1/4 cup red onion, cut into chunks
- 1 tablespoon olive oil
- Seasonings (oregano, paprika, salt, and pepper to taste)

Instructions:

1. In a bowl, mix shrimp with seasonings.
2. Thread shrimp and vegetables onto skewers.
3. Brush with olive oil and grill until shrimp are cooked.

Nutritional value (approx. per serving):

- Calories. 200
- Protein. 25g
- Carbohydrates. 8g
- Fiber. 3g

Prep. Time: 30 minutes (includes grilling)

54. RecllBaked Cod with Tomato Salsa

Ingredients:

- 2 cod filets (6 oz each)

- 1/2 cup diced tomatoes
- 1/4 cup diced onions
- 1/4 cup diced bell peppers
- 1/4 cup chopped cilantro
- 1 tablespoon olive oil
- Lime juice, to taste

Instructions:
1. Preheat the oven to 375°F (190°C).
2. Season cod filets with salt, pepper, and olive oil.
3. Combine diced tomatoes, onions, bell peppers, cilantro, and lime juice.
4. Spoon the salsa over the cod.
5. Bake until the cod is cooked through.

Nutritional value (approx. per serving):
- Calories. 250
- Protein. 30g
- Carbohydrates. 10g
- Fiber. 3g

Prep. Time: 25 minutes

55. Lemon Garlic Shrimp Scampi

Ingredients:
- 8 oz (225g) large shrimp, peeled and deveined
- 2 tablespoons olive oil
- 3 cloves garlic, minced

- 1 lemon, juiced and zested
- Fresh parsley for garnish
- Whole wheat pasta (optional)

Instructions:

1. In a pan, heat olive oil and sauté minced garlic.
2. Add shrimp and cook until pink.
3. Stir in lemon juice and zest.
4. Serve over whole wheat pasta or with a side of vegetables.

Nutritional Value (approx. per serving without pasta):

- Calories. 180
- Protein. 25g
- Carbohydrates. 3g
- Fiber. 0g

Prep. Time: 20 minutes

56. Tuna Salad with Greek Yogurt

Ingredients:
- 1 can (5 oz) canned tuna, drained
- 1/2 cup low-fat Greek yogurt
- 1/4 cup diced celery
- 1/4 cup diced red onion
- 1 tablespoon fresh dill
- Salt and pepper to taste
- Whole wheat crackers (for serving)

Instructions:
1. In a bowl, combine drained tuna, Greek yogurt, celery, red onion, and dill.
2. Season with salt and pepper.
3. Serve with whole wheat crackers or on whole wheat bread.

Nutritional Value (approx. for salad without crackers):
- Calories. 200
- Protein. 25g
- Carbohydrates. 10g
- Fiber. 2g

Prep. Time: 10 minutes

56. Lemon Herb Baked Tilapia

Ingredients:

- 2 tilapia filets (6 oz each)
- 1 lemon, juiced and zested
- 1 tablespoon fresh herbs (rosemary, thyme, or your choice)
- Salt and pepper to taste
- Olive oil for drizzling

Instructions:

1. Preheat the oven to 375°F (190°C).
2. Season tilapia filets with lemon zest, herbs, salt, and pepper.
3. Drizzle with lemon juice and olive oil.
4. Bake until tilapia is cooked through.

Nutritional value (approx. per serving):

- Calories. 150
- Protein. 30g
- Carbohydrates. 2g
- Fiber. 0g

Prep. Time: 20 minutes

57. Garlic Butter Shrimp and Asparagus

Ingredients:
- 8 oz (225g) large shrimp, peeled and deveined
- 1 bunch asparagus, trimmed
- 3 tablespoons butter
- 3 cloves garlic, minced
- Lemon wedges

Instructions:
1. In a pan, melt butter and sauté minced garlic.
2. Add shrimp and cook until pink.
3. Add asparagus and cook until tender.
4. Serve with lemon wedges.

Nutritional value (approx. per serving):
- Calories. 250
- Protein. 25g
- Carbohydrates. 6g
- Fiber. 3g

Prep. Time: 20 minutes

58. Grilled Swordfish with Mango Salsa

Ingredients:
- 2 swordfish steaks (6 oz each)
- 1 ripe mango, diced
- 1/4 cup red onion, finely chopped
- 1/4 cup chopped cilantro
- 1 lime, juiced and zested
- Salt and pepper to taste

Instructions:
1. Season swordfish with salt and pepper.
2. Grill swordfish until cooked through.
3. In a bowl, combine diced mango, red onion, cilantro, lime juice, and zest.
4. Serve grilled swordfish with mango salsa.

Nutritional value (approx. per serving):
- Calories. 300
- Protein. 30g
- Carbohydrates. 15g
- Fiber. 2g

Preparation Time: 30 minutes

59. Spicy Baked Catfish

Ingredients
- 2 catfish filets (6 oz each)
- 2 tablespoons olive oil
- 1 teaspoon paprika
- 1/2 teaspoon cayenne pepper (adjust to taste)
- 1/2 teaspoon garlic powder
- Lemon wedges

Instructions:
1. Preheat the oven to 375°F (190°C).
2. In a bowl, mix olive oil, paprika, cayenne pepper, and garlic powder.
3. Brush the catfish filets with the spice mixture.
4. Bake until the catfish is cooked through.
5. Serve with lemon wedges.

Nutritional value (approx. per serving):
- Calories. 280
- Protein. 25g
- Carbohydrates. 3g
- Fiber. 1g

Prep. Time: 25 minutes

60. Garlic Butter Scallop Scampi

Ingredients:
- 8 oz (225g) scallops
- 3 tablespoons butter
- 4 cloves garlic, minced
- 1/4 cup white wine (or chicken broth)
- Lemon wedges
- Fresh parsley for garnish
- Whole wheat pasta (optional)

Instructions:
1. In a pan, melt butter and sauté minced garlic.
2. Add scallops and cook until they are opaque.
3. Pour in white wine (or chicken broth) and simmer until reduced.
4. Serve over whole wheat pasta or with a side of vegetables.
5. Garnish with lemon wedges and fresh parsley.

Nutritional Value (approx. per serving without pasta).
- Calories. 200
- Protein. 20g
- Carbohydrates. 3g
- Fiber. 0g

Prep. Time: 20 minutes

CHAPTER 10

61. Roasted Vegetable Medley

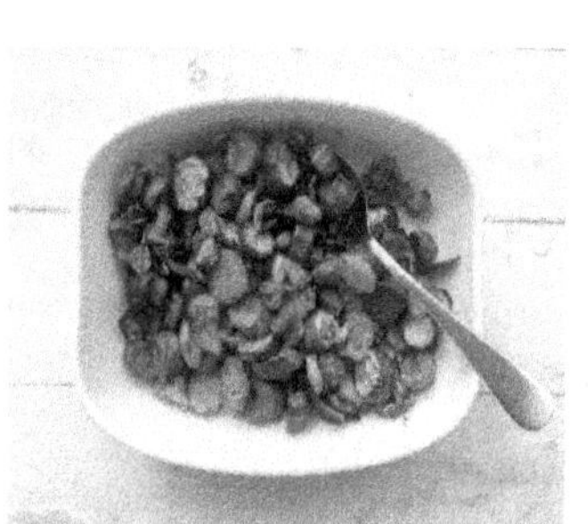

Nutritional value (approx. per serving):
- Calories. 100
- Carbohydrates. 12g
- Fiber. 3g

Prep. Time: 30 minutes (includes roasting)

Ingredients:

- 2 cups mixed vegetables (zucchini, bell peppers, cherry tomatoes, carrots)
- 2 tablespoons olive oil
- Seasonings (rosemary, thyme, garlic powder)
- Salt and pepper to taste

Instructions:

1. Preheat the oven to 400°F (200°C).
2. Toss mixed vegetables with olive oil, seasonings, salt, and pepper.
3. Spread them on a baking sheet and roast until tender.

62. Spinach and Mushroom Salad

Ingredients:
- 2 cups fresh spinach leaves
- 1 cup sliced mushrooms
- 1/4 cup diced red onion
- 2 tablespoons balsamic vinegar
- 1 tablespoon olive oil
- Salt and pepper to taste

Instructions:
1. In a salad bowl, combine spinach, mushrooms, and red onion.
2. In a small bowl, whisk balsamic vinegar, olive oil, salt, and pepper.
3. Drizzle the dressing over the salad.

Nutritional value (approx. per serving):
- Calories. 80
- Carbohydrates. 8g
- Fiber. 2g

Prep. Time: 10 minutes

63. Steamed Broccoli with Lemon Butter

Ingredients:
- 2 cups broccoli florets
- 2 tablespoons unsalted butter
- 1 lemon, juiced and zested
- Salt and pepper to taste

Instructions:
1. Steam the broccoli until tender.
2. In a small saucepan, melt butter and mix with lemon juice and zest.
3. Drizzle the lemon butter over the steamed broccoli.

Nutritional value (approx. per serving):
- Calories. 100
- Carbohydrates. 10g
- Fiber. 4g

Prep. Time: 15 minutes (includes steaming)

64. Cucumber and Tomato Salad

Ingredients:
- 1 cucumber, sliced
- 1 cup cherry tomatoes, halved
- 1/4 cup red onion, thinly sliced
- 2 tablespoons fresh basil, chopped
- 1 tablespoon olive oil
- Balsamic vinegar to taste
- Salt and pepper to taste

Instructions:
1. In a salad bowl, combine cucumber, cherry tomatoes, red onion, and fresh basil.
2. Drizzle with olive oil and balsamic vinegar. Season with salt and pepper.

Nutritional value (approx. per serving):
- Calories. 80
- Carbohydrates. 10g
- Fiber. 2g

Prep. Time: 10 minutes

65. Sautéed Asparagus with Garlic

Ingredients:
- 2 cups asparagus spears, trimmed
- 2 cloves garlic, minced
- 1 tablespoon olive oil
- Lemon wedges

Instructions:

1. In a pan, sauté asparagus with minced garlic in olive oil until tender.

2. Serve with lemon wedges.

Nutritional value (approx. per serving):
- Calories. 70
- Carbohydrates. 7g
- Fiber. 3g

Prep. Time: 15 minutes

66. Sweet Potato Mash

Ingredients:

- 2 medium sweet potatoes, peeled and diced
- 2 tablespoons Greek yogurt
- 1 tablespoon honey (optional)
- Cinnamon to taste

Instructions:

1. Boil or steam sweet potatoes until soft.
2. Mash them and mix with Greek yogurt, honey (if desired), and cinnamon.

Nutritional value (approx. per serving):

- Calories. 150
- Carbohydrates. 30g
- Fiber. 4g

Preparation Time: 20 minutes (includes boiling)

67. Grilled Eggplant with Pesto

Ingredients:
- 2 slices of eggplant
- 2 tablespoons homemade or store-bought pesto sauce
- Olive oil for grilling
- Fresh basil leaves for garnish

Instructions:
1. Brush eggplant slices with olive oil and grill until tender.
2. Spread pesto sauce on grilled eggplant slices.
3. Garnish with fresh basil leaves.

Nutritional value (approx. per serving):
- Calories. 120
- Carbohydrates. 7g
- Fiber. 3g

Prep. Time: 15 minutes (includes grilling).

68. Stir-Fried Bok Choy

Ingredients:
- 2 cups bok choy, chopped
- 1 clove garlic, minced
- 1 tablespoon low-sodium soy sauce
- 1 tablespoon olive oil
- Sesame seeds for garnish

Instructions:
1. In a wok, sauté minced garlic in olive oil.
2. Add bok choy and stir-fry until wilted.
3. Drizzle with low-sodium soy sauce and garnish with sesame seeds.

Nutritional value (approx. per serving):
- Calories. 70
- Carbohydrates. 5g
- Fiber. 2g

Prep. Time: 10 minutes

69. Butternut Squash Soup

Ingredients:
- 2 cups diced butternut squash
- 1/2 cup diced onion
- 1 clove garlic, minced
- 4 cups low-sodium chicken or vegetable broth
- 1 teaspoon fresh thyme
- Salt and pepper to taste

Instructions:
1. In a pot, sauté diced onion and minced garlic until translucent.
2. Add butternut squash, thyme, and broth.
3. Simmer until squash is tender, then blend until smooth.
4. Season with salt and pepper.

Nutritional value (approx. per serving):
- Calories. 120
- Carbohydrates. 30g
- Fiber. 5g

Prep. Time: 30 minutes

70. Grilled Portobello Mushrooms

Ingredients:
- 2 portobello mushrooms
- 2 tablespoons balsamic vinegar
- 1 tablespoon olive oil
- Fresh basil leaves for garnish

Instructions:
1. Brush portobello mushrooms with olive oil and balsamic vinegar
2. Grill until tender
3. Garnish with
4. fresh basil leaves

Nutritional value (approx. per serving):
- Calories. 70
- Carbohydrates. 6g
- Fiber. 2g

Prep. Time: 15 minutes (includes grilling)

CHAPTER 11

DESSERT

71. Greek Yogurt with Berries

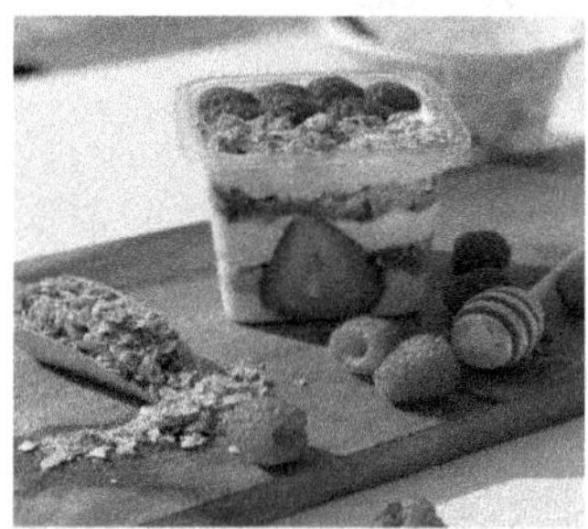

Nutritional value.
(approx. per serving).
Calories. 150
Protein. 10g
Carbs. 20g
Fiber. 3g
Prep. Time:5 minutes

Ingredients:

- 1 cup low-fat Greek yogurt
- 1/2 cup blended berries (blueberries, strawberries, raspberries)
- 1 tablespoon honey (discretionary)

Instructions:

1. In a bowl, join Greek yogurt and blended berries.
2. Shower with honey whenever wanted.

72. Prepared Apples with Cinnamon

Ingredients:
- 2 medium apples
- 1/2 teaspoon ground cinnamon
- 1 tablespoon honey (discretionary)
- 1/4 cup hacked pecans

Instructions:
1. Preheat the stove to 375°F (190°C).
2. Center the apples and sprinkle with cinnamon.
3. Shower with honey and top with slashed pecans.
4. Prepare until the apples are delicate and delicate.

- **Nutritional value. (approx. per serving).**
  - Calories. 200
  - Protein. 2g
  - Carbs. 30g
  - Fiber. 5g

Prep. Time:30 minutes (counting baking)

73. Chia Pudding with Almond Milk

Ingredients:

- 2 tablespoons chia seeds
- 1 cup unsweetened almond milk
- 1/2 teaspoon vanilla concentrate
- New berries for fixing

Instructions:

1. In a bowl, consolidate chia seeds, almond milk, and vanilla concentrate.

2. Mix well, cover, and refrigerate for a couple of hours or short-term until it thickens.

3. Top with new berries prior to serving.

Nutritional value (approx. per serving).
- Calories. 150
- Protein. 4g
- Starches. 10g
- Fiber. 8g

Prep. Time:5 minutes (in addition to chilling time)

74. Banana and Pecan Oatmeal

Ingredients:
- 1/2 cup dated oats
- 1 cup unsweetened almond milk
- 1 ready banana, pounded
- 2 tablespoons slashed pecans
- Cinnamon to taste

Instructions:
1. In a pot, consolidate oats and almond milk.
2. Cook over medium intensity until oats are delicate and combination thickens.
3. Mix in pounded banana, slashed pecans, and cinnamon.

Nutritional value (approx. per serving).
- Calories. 250
- Protein. 6g
- Sugars. 40g
- Fiber. 6g

Prep. Time:15 minutes

75. Berry Parfait with Yogurt

Ingredients:
- 1 cup low-fat plain yogurt
- 1/2 cup blended berries (strawberries, blueberries, raspberries)
- 1/4 cup granola (pick a low-sugar choice)

Instructions:
1. In a glass, layer yogurt, blended berries, and granola.
2. Rehash the layers.
3. Top with a couple of berries.

Nutritional value (approx. per serving).
- Calories. 200
- Protein. 8g
- Sugars. 30g
- Fiber. 5g

Prep. Time:5 minutes

76. Organic product Salad with Mint

Ingredients:

- 1 cup blended organic product (pineapple, melon, grapes)
- 1 tablespoon new mint leaves, cleaved
- 1/2 lime, squeezed
- 1/2 teaspoon honey (discretionary)

Instructions:

1. In a bowl, join blended products of the soil mint.
2. Sprinkle it with lime squeeze and honey whenever you want.

Nutritional value (approx. per serving).
- Calories. 80
- Protein. 1g
- Sugars. 20g
- Fiber. 2g

Prep. Time: 10 minutes

77. Rice Pudding with Cinnamon

Ingredients:

- 1/2 cup cooked earthy colored rice
- 1 cup unsweetened almond milk
- 1/2 teaspoon ground cinnamon
- 1/4 teaspoon vanilla concentrate
- 1 tablespoon raisins

Instructions:

1. In a pot, consolidate cooked rice and almond milk.
2. Cook over low intensity until it thickens.
3. Mix in cinnamon, vanilla concentrate, and raisins.

Nutritional value (approx. per serving).
- Calories. 180
- Protein. 4g
- Sugars. 35g
- Fiber. 3g

Prep. Time: 15 minutes

78. Blended Berry Sorbet

Ingredients:
- 2 cups blended frozen berries (strawberries, blueberries, raspberries)
- 1/4 cup unsweetened squeezed apple
- 1 tablespoon honey (discretionary)

Instructions:
1. In a blender, join frozen berries, squeezed apple, and honey (whenever wanted).
2. Mix until smooth.
3. Freeze for a couple of hours until firm.

Nutritional value. (approx. per serving).
- Calories. 120
- Protein. 1g
- Carbs. 30g
- Fiber. 5g

Prep. Time:10 minutes (in addition to freezing time)

79. Almond and Date Energy Balls

Ingredients:

- 1 cup almonds
- 1/2 cup pitted dates
- 1/4 cup unsweetened cocoa powder
- 1 teaspoon vanilla concentrate
- A touch of salt

Instructions:

1. In a food processor, consolidate almonds, dates, cocoa powder, vanilla concentrate, and a touch of salt.
2. Process until the blend remains together.
3. Structure into little balls and refrigerate.

Nutritional value (approx. per serving).
- Calories. 120
- Protein. 3g
- Sugars. 15g
- Fiber. 3g

Prep. Time: 15 minutes

80. Avocado Chocolate Mousse

Ingredients:
- 2 ready avocados
- 1/4 cup unsweetened cocoa powder
- 1/4 cup honey (or to taste)
- 1/2 teaspoon vanilla concentrate

Instructions:
1. In a blender, join avocados, cocoa powder, honey, and vanilla concentrate.
2. Mix until smooth and velvety.
3. Chill in the fridge prior to serving.

Nutritional value (approx. per serving).
- Calories. 150
- Protein. 2g
- Starches. 20g
- Fiber. 7g

Prep. Time:10 minutes (in addition to chilling time).

RECOMMENDED WORKOUT

- **Energetic strolling**. Lively strolling is an extraordinary method for beginning with oxygen consuming activity. Go for the golden 30 minutes of energetic strolling most days of the week.

- **Running or Jogging**. Running and jogging are more extreme types of oxygen consuming activity that can assist with consuming more calories. In the event that you are new to running or running, begin gradually and step by step increment the span and force of your exercises.

- **Swimming**. Swimming is an extraordinary low-influence practice that is kind with the joints. An extraordinary choice for individuals are overweight or stout.

- **Cycling**. Cycling is an incredible method for getting cardiovascular activity while likewise partaking in the outside.

- **Moving**. Moving is a tomfoolery and a viable method for getting exercise. It is an incredible method for consuming calories and working on your coordination.

- **Strength preparing works out**. Strength preparing activities like weightlifting, bodyweight activities, and obstruction band activities can assist with building muscle. Muscle assists consume calories, which with canning assist with diminishing liver fat.

In the event that you have any worries about beginning an activity program, converse with your PCP. They can assist you with making a protected and viable activity plan that is ideal for you.

CONCLUSION

This Fatty Liver diet Cookbook fills in as a thorough manual for changing your dietary propensities and assuming responsibility for your wellbeing. Fatty liver sickness is a quiet plague that can have serious results, yet through the cautious choice of recipes and fixings presented in this book, you can leave on an excursion toward recuperation and generally prosperity.

All through these pages, we've investigated heavenly, supplement stuffed recipes that help liver wellbeing as well as entice your taste buds. The accentuation on entire food sources, lean proteins, and plant-based choices gives a decent way to deal with sustaining your body and forestalling the movement of greasy liver sickness.

As you leave this culinary experience, recall that your wellbeing is your most valuable resource. By embracing the standards illustrated in this cookbook, you're moving toward mending and revival. The force of nourishment couldn't possibly be more significant, and your decisions in the kitchen are an immediate impression of your obligation to a better, more joyful life.

In this way, let the fragrance of these nutritious dishes fill your kitchen, and the flavors animate your sense of taste. As you enjoy each nibble, imagine your liver recuperating and your body flourishing. This cookbook is something beyond an assortment of recipes; it's an extraordinary device for working on your personal satisfaction.

In your excursion towards a better you, recollect that change takes time, commitment, and constancy. It's not generally simple, however the prizes are endless. Give this cookbook to your friend to access your mission for better wellbeing. Share your triumphs, gain from your difficulties, and remain persuaded. You deserve it and your friends and family to earnestly embrace this excursion.

Eventually, your wellbeing is your most significant inspiration. Embrace this cookbook, relish the advantages of a liver-accommodating eating regimen, and watch your prosperity thrive. You have the ability to have an effect in your life, each dinner in turn. Bon appétit and all the best on your way to a better, more joyful you.

28-Day Meal Plan

DAYS	BREAKFAST	LUNCH	SNACKS	DINNER
1.	Avocado and Spinach Breakfast Bowl	Grilled Chicken and Vegetable Salad	Hard-Boiled Eggs	Baked Salmon with Asparagus
2.	Greek Yogurt Parfait	Quinoa and Black Bean Salad	Apple Slices with Almond Butter	Turkey and Vegetable Stir-Fry
3.	Oatmeal with Berries and Almonds	Lentil and Vegetable Soup	Mixed Nuts	Grilled Chicken with Roasted Vegetables
4.	Spinach and Mushroom Omelette	Tuna and White Bean Salad	Cucumber and Hummus	Lentil and Spinach Curry
5.	Quinoa and Fruit Breakfast	Baked Salmon with	Greek Yogurt and Berry	Quinoa and Black Bean Stuffed

	Bowl	Roasted Vegetables	Parfait	Peppers
6.	Sweet Potato Hash	Quinoa and Roasted Vegetable Bowl	Cottage Cheese with Pineapple	Shrimp and Broccoli Quinoa Bowl
7.	Chia Seed Pudding	Shrimp and Broccoli Stir-Fry	Berry and Spinach Smoothie	Tofu and Vegetable Stir-Fry
10.	Banana and Almond Butter Toast	Spinach and Feta Stuffed Chicken Breast	Sliced Bell Peppers with Guacamole	Lemon Herb Baked Chicken
11.	Cottage Cheese and Berries Bowl	Turkey and Avocado Wrap	Whole Wheat Toast with Avocado	Baked Cod with Salsa
12.	Veggie and Egg Breakfast	Chickpea and Cucumber	Carrot and Hummus	Eggplant and Lentil Stew

	Wrap	Salad		
13.	Cottage Cheese and Berries Bowl	Grilled chicken breast with quinoa salad	Almonds and a piece of fruit St ir-fried tofu with	Stir-fried tofu with vegetables
14.	Whole grain toast with avocado	Fruit smoothie with spinach and banana	Cherry tomatoes with mozzarell a Le an beef stir-fry with	Baked cod with a side of brown rice
15.	Greek yogurt with honey and walnuts	Tuna salad on whole wheat bread	Mixed nuts and dried fruits	Lean beef stir-fry with broccoli
16.	Fruit smoothie with spinach and banana	Grilled vegetable wrap with whole grain	Sliced cucumber s with tzatziki dip Gr illed portobello	Grilled turkey burger with sweet potatoes

No.				
17.	Whole grain cereal with low-fat milk	Spinach and feta stuffed chicken breast	Celery and peanut butter	Lean beef stir-fry with broccoli
18.	Avocado and tomato omelet	Quinoa and Roasted Vegetable Bowl	Hard-Boiled Eggs	Baked Salmon with Asparagus
19.	Cottage Cheese and Berries Bowl	Chickpea and Cucumber Salad	Carrot and Hummus	Turkey and Vegetable Stir-Fry
20.	Banana and Almond Butter Toast	Fruit smoothie with spinach and banana	Almonds and a piece of fruit St ir-fried tofu with	Lemon Herb Baked Chicken
21.	Veggie and Egg Breakfast Wrap	Grilled vegetable wrap with whole grain	Celery and peanut butter	Grilled turkey burger with sweet potatoes

22.	Greek yogurt	Spinach and feta	Sliced cucumb	Grilled turkey

	with honey and walnuts	stuffed chicken breast	ers with tzatziki dip Grilled portobello	burger with sweet potatoes
23.	Whole grain toast with avocado	Grilled chicken breast with quinoa salad	Almonds and a piece of fruit Stir-fried tofu with	Eggplant and Lentil Stew
24.	Cottage Cheese and Berries Bowl	Tuna salad on whole wheat bread	Cherry tomatoes with mozzarella Lean beef stir-fry with	Stir-fried tofu with vegetables
25.	Spinach and Mushroom Omelette	Tuna salad on whole wheat bread	Celery and peanut butter	Turkey and Vegetable Stir-Fry

26.	Veggie and Egg Breakfast Wrap	Grilled vegetable wrap with whole grain	Mixed nuts and dried fruits	Baked Cod with Salsa
27.	Avocado and Spinach Breakfast Bowl	Grilled chicken breast with quinoa salad	Cherry tomatoes with mozzarella Lean beef stir-fry with	Stir-fried tofu with vegetables
28.	Cottage Cheese and Berries Bowl	Spinach and feta stuffed chicken breast	Mixed nuts and dried fruits	Grilled turkey burger with sweet potatoes